# Type 2 Diabetes:

# From diagnosis to a new way of life

## Matthew Lashley

# Disclaimer

This book is not intended as a substitute for the medical advice of physicians. The reader should regularly consult a physician in matters relating to his/her health and particularly with respect to any symptoms that may require diagnosis or medical attention.

# Table of Contents

Acknowledgments i

1 From denial to self-blame Pg 1

2 Acceptance Pg 9

3 A serious illness Pg 13

4 Gaining control Pg 17

5 Daily calorie target levels Pg 23

6 Foods to eat and avoid Pg 29

7 The importance of fiber Pg 35

8 No more sweets? Pg 41

9 Eating out at restaurants Pg 45

10 Is type 2 diabetes reversible? Pg 51

A Last Word

Helpful Resources

# ACKNOWLEDGMENTS

I wrote this book to help others, but I would not be here today without the support of my family and friends who encouraged me to fight this disease. Above all, I must thank my daughter. Although I suffered a deep depression for weeks after my diagnosis, she encouraged me daily to take control over my condition and not let it dictate the future of my life.

# Chapter 1

## From denial to self-blame

It started with a nose infection. I don't know how it happened, but I had a nostril begin to swell and in a matter of 48 hours, my entire face was swollen. With no time to make an appointment with a doctor and not wanting to go to a walk-in emergency room, I made an appointment at a local clinic. I was able to get in the same day I called and was examined by a physicians assistant or PA. He prescribed an anti-biotic that cleared up my infection, but while I was being examined, he noticed that my blood pressure was high. Since I hadn't had any blood work done in many years, he thought it best for me to have blood testing done and to see a doctor for a check-up. I agreed. I had some medical issues that seemed to be getting worse and wanted to talk to a doctor about them. Specifically, I was feeling numbness in my lower legs and feet. Since my late teens, I have experienced an issue with a herniated disc on the lower left side of my back. This has created pain that comes and goes. Lately, however, the pain was replaced by numbness. What was alarming to me was that this numbness was in both legs. I had experienced numbness before in the left leg, but it always was due to the way I was sitting and crossing my legs. Simply standing up would make the numbness go away. Now, it was as if my left foot and lower leg were in a state of between normal and falling asleep. This feeling had now spread to my right leg and foot, so I feared that I would need back surgery. There were a few other issues that I wanted to mention to the doctor. I was having problems with my eyesight, and I had a couple of cuts on my arm that were not healing right. Of course, there was the issue of high blood pressure.

I began taking my blood pressure with a battery operated machine I had at home. After three weeks of testing, I was averaging 137/82. I didn't think this was too bad, but I wrote down the data for the doctor. A few days after going to the test lab for blood work, I went to the doctor. I took a short list of my medical issues, so I would remember to ask about everything. There was a nurse that took my blood pressure and another nurse that took some data on my heart rate. Other basic information was taken such as weight and pulse rate. I waited for the doctor and was thinking about which one of my medical problems I was going to ask about first. I decided on the blood pressure problem.

The doctor came in the room, sat down in front of a computer screen to look at my test results, and I handed her the sheet of paper showing all of the data from three weeks of blood pressure readings. She took a moment to look at the readings, and then asked me if anyone had spoken to me about my test results. I replied, no. The doctor then looked at me in the eyes and said, "You have diabetes."

I replied, "I don't think so." I didn't realize what I was saying. I was disagreeing with a medical doctor. She repeated, "You have diabetes." Clearly she was not going to argue with me, but I told her that maybe they mislabeled the urine sample.

Although there seemed to be a protocol followed with the blood sample, I simply handed a technician the urine sample at the test lab. She informed me that my glucose level came from the blood sample. After an eight hour fast, my glucose level should be between 70 and 100. My number of 287 was entirely too high. She left the room and had a nurse check my glucose level with a hand held meter. At that moment it was 327, and this was alarming because it was at least two hours after breakfast, and I was hungry.

When the doctor came back, I told her about my back problem and the numbness in my legs. After taking my socks off, she stuck my toes with a pin. I felt nothing. It wasn't my back. The condition was called neuropathy, and it was due to high levels of glucose in my blood for a prolonged period of time. Suddenly, I became aware that all of my medical issues were only symptoms of one medical condition: I was a type 2 diabetic. She gave me a prescription for a basic medication for type 2 diabetes and even a prescription for my elevated blood pressure although this may have been related to glucose levels. I was given a name and number of an organization to call for education and assistance with my medical condition.

I walked out of the doctor's office still in a state of shock. How can I be a type 2 diabetic? Everybody knows that this is a problem that comes from bad eating habits. Only the obese get type 2 diabetes. At 5'11", I only weighed 155 pounds. I wasn't overweight. In fact, I was a little on the skinny side. My mother was a type 2 diabetic, but she was also overweight and ate a lot of sweets. It was understandable that she became a diabetic, but why me? I took good care of myself.

My doctor gave me a glucose meter and a nurse showed me how to use it. With a prescription for diabetic medication and test strips, I stopped by the local pharmacy to get a supply of medication and test strips then went home with my meter. I was still skeptical about having type 2 diabetes, but with an engineering background and a meter, I was willing to take blood glucose measurements, record my readings and visit the doctor for a follow-up examination.

Because of my mother, I understood the basic diet for a type 2 diabetic. Basically it was a low carbohydrate diet, but I decided to only eliminate the sweets from my diet. Surely that was my only problem. The donut in the morning with my coffee and perhaps an afternoon candy bar were eliminated. Without eating these things, my sugar levels did drop down, but not enough to be close to normal and still high enough to be dangerous to my health. I had made some progress in lowering my sugar levels, but it was clear that it wasn't enough. I had type 2 diabetes, and in order to get it under control, I needed to accept this.

## How I found out what Type 2 diabetes was

My mother needed emergency assistance, and the paramedics were called to help her. She couldn't breathe. The rest of the family thought it was her heart, but the paramedics didn't think so. Her heart was normal as well as her blood pressure; however, her blood sugar was very high, and they wanted to know what her normal readings were like. I didn't know that she was a diabetic at the time. I remember in grade school having a friend who was a diabetic and he took insulin shots every day. This was because his pancreas did not produce enough insulin for his body. The paramedic told me that it was a different kind of diabetes. My mother apparently had type 2 diabetes. This was a condition when the body builds up a tolerance for insulin and doesn't process it as efficiently. This was the first explanation of type 2 diabetes that I had ever heard. One of the problems that can happen with high blood sugar is a stroke. After they took her to the hospital, it was later discovered that it was a stroke that she had experienced.

# Chapter 2

## Acceptance and getting down to work

If there is one thing that I learned that helped me to accept my medical condition, it was to understand that it was not my fault that I had type 2 diabetes. Too often, you will hear conversations about people with type 2 diabetes as if they are responsible for their own condition. You can even hear this on radio and television programs. Sometimes it will be doctors that say this. It simply is not true. I was one of these people, and this was one of the reasons I was in denial. It is only the obese that get diabetes and perhaps those that eat too much sugar. Of course, the truth is most people who are overweight are not diabetics. In the future, scientific research into this area may yield good information and help to prevent this disease, but for now, it is only important that you accept this medical condition in your life and take action to reduce its effect on your health.

# Medication

I was prescribed Metformin from the beginning. This is a medication that works on the liver to suppress glucose. The liver has many functions and one of them is to store glucose so that it will be available when the body needs extra amounts. A type 2 diabetic has plenty of glucose in the blood; the problem is that insulin is not breaking down the glucose quick enough. This medication is a standard prescription for those who are recently diagnosed with type 2 diabetes. The idea is to start using this medication and see how well glucose levels could be controlled with diet and exercise.

I became motivated to work as hard as possible to control my glucose because the possibilities with drugs are limited and there are many side effects. In some cases, insulin can be used, but the body is already intolerant of insulin. I knew that increasing insulin in a type 2 diabetic can be dangerous. Simply looking at my mother and her diet, I could see the danger. A high carbohydrate diet that included many sweets required insulin injected into the blood, but the first time she went without a meal or sugary snacks, it was possible for her sugar levels to drop below normal. When this happens, a person can slip into a coma. By controlling my type 2 diabetes primarily with diet and exercise, I knew I would not have to worry about low blood sugar and only focus on the high end of my glucose readings.

# Chapter 3

## Type 2 diabetes is a serious illness

Even those who realize they have type 2 diabetes often do not understand how serious of an illness this is. Left alone, diabetes will kill you. Unfortunately, it is a silent killer. Symptoms may not be apparent, but over time damage to your body will accumulate resulting in the failure of your kidneys or a deadly stroke. Others may suffer several symptoms of diabetes that slowly grind away at their health until one day death occurs, and the only way to categorize the cause of death is with the general statement of, "complications due to diabetes". If you are someone who has been diagnosed with type 2 diabetes but does not yet have any major symptoms, you should consider yourself lucky. Many people find out after a great deal of damage has been done. I have the condition known as neuropathy. This means that I have sustained nerve damage from high levels of glucose over an extended period of time. This has resulted in numbness in my legs below the knee and extending to my feet. Although I cannot feel my toes, I can still wiggle them, so I have enough nerve function that I can walk. I consider myself lucky.

## The silent killer

Type 2 diabetes is a deadly disease, and it could kill you tomorrow, next week, or slowly destroy you piece by piece. There is no way to predict the exact health problems that type 2 diabetes will create to take your life, but sooner or later, it will. Having a stroke is one of the leading causes of death, but kidney failure ranks high as well. Type 2 diabetes can take away your vision as well as your legs. It can cause hypertension and cause death from conditions related to high blood pressure. There may even be a link between diabetes and dementia. Often an individual with type 2 diabetes will not suffer much from the symptoms and doesn't do anything about the condition, but diabetes often creeps upon a person in silence. If you wait until something serious happens to you, it may be too late to recover. The good news is that you can take steps to control your diabetes, and greatly increase the chances of longevity.

# Chapter 4

## Gaining control over blood glucose levels

My first glucose fasting test produced a number of 287, but six months later it was well under 100 at a nice 94. Looking at this number alone, a doctor could easily conclude that I was not a diabetic. Or maybe I have been cured of diabetes. Of course, this is absurd. I not only take medication, but most importantly, I have spent months sticking to a low carbohydrate diet within limits that keeps my glucose at less than dangerous levels. My 100 grams of carbohydrates per day keeps my average glucose level down, but the fact is, my numbers still spike higher than a normal person's blood sugar does. After a big meal, I can easily hit the mid 160s. Equally important is the fact that my glucose levels drop more slowly than a non-diabetic. Exercise, of course, has played an important part in keeping my glucose levels down. My goal is to keep my glucose levels to as close to normal as possible and keep my body from deteriorating any more than it already has from high glucose levels in the blood.

## Sugary foods and snacks

When people think of diabetes, they think of sugary foods, but in truth, it is the carbohydrates that will raise your blood sugar. The only difference between a nutritional food high in carbohydrates and a sugary snack like a candy bar is the candy bar will produce a spike in blood sugar more quickly. For this reason alone, it can be more dangerous because a high enough blood sugar spike can cause a stroke. Fortunately, you don't have to be concerned about sugar intake because gram for gram, sugary foods are higher in carbohydrates than nutritional foods. By limiting your carbohydrate intake to a certain number, you will find yourself automatically eliminating sugary snacks to adhere to a daily carbohydrate budget.

## How many carbohydrates per day should the limit be?

Only you with the help of your doctor can determine this. The key to finding out what your daily carbohydrate limit should be is testing your blood. After every meal or snack, write down the number of grams of carbohydrates you have consumed. If possible, you should do this before you eat, so you will know if you are about to eat too many grams of carbohydrates. When you check your blood sugar one to two hours after eating, you need to record the number. Take a few quick notes about how many grams of carbohydrates you ate and what you ate. Try and spread the total daily carbohydrates into three separate meals. After a few weeks, you will know what your limit is to get your glucose numbers down as well as what you need to limit yourself to after obtaining your goals.

Starting at levels of over 300, I found that I was able to

reduce my glucose levels quickly with a limit of 60 – 80 grams of carbohydrates each day. It took several weeks to get my numbers down, but once I was able to reach my desired glucose target numbers, I was able to maintain them at 100 grams of carbohydrates each day.

## My target glucose levels

The amount of carbohydrate grams you are looking to limit your daily intake to will be directly related to the glucose numbers that you are trying to obtain in your blood. These numbers are something you should consult your doctor about; however, many doctors are not as familiar with type 2 diabetes as other doctors are and may not provide the guidance you need. If this is the case, then begin with the numbers provided by the American Diabetes Association. Their general guidelines are as follows:

Less than 130 before you eat

Less than 180 two hours after a meal

Less than 140 before you go to bed

These were the numbers I used in the beginning when attempting to lower my blood sugar with one exception and that is the 130 number before eating. My glucose reading had been 287 after fasting. In order to get below 130 before a meal, I would have to starve myself to the point I would be admitted to an emergency room. So I focused on the after meal spikes and tried to get it below 180. I checked my blood after each meal and reduced by carbohydrate intake. I took more than two months, but I was able to get the after meal spikes below 180. At this point, I was able to monitor my before meal number and hold it under 130.

## The dawn phenomenon

One problem I discovered as I attempted to lower my blood sugar level was that my number rose sometime during the night. I could go to bed with a certain glucose number, and in the morning, it would be higher. This is without eating anything. I never understood what was happening, and it didn't seem there was a clear explanation from the medical community. I do know that I am not the only one to experience this problem. There are many who have discussed this in forums on the Internet. In fact, that is where I first read the term dawn phenomenon. It is a real problem, and the only thing I could do was to avoid eating my dinner late at night, so I would go to bed with a reasonable glucose number. Now that I have my glucose under control, I don't worry about a minor spike in glucose during the night because I go to bed with a low enough glucose level that I will not be in any danger.

# Chapter 5

## Daily calorie target levels compliment glucose target levels

I found out quickly that I needed to keep my calorie intake to a level that my body required to operate. I wasn't overweight when I was diagnosed with type 2 diabetes, but I did have a little fat on me. At 5'11" I weighed 155 pounds. My typical intake of calories for the day to maintain my weight, doing a moderate amount of exercise, was about 2000. When I went over this for the day, I found that my glucose numbers would begin to creep up. The same was true for a meal. Large meals of over 700 calories, even if they were low in carbohydrates, would still make my sugar go up. Of course, it wasn't as dramatic as with high carbohydrate foods, but testing my blood sugar made it clear that I not only needed to keep my carbohydrates down, but watch my weight as well. Since my first diagnosis, I now weigh 150, but this is as low as my weight can go without becoming unhealthy. Being overweight may or may not have anything to do with developing diabetes, but losing weight can be an important tool in lowering blood glucose levels. Keeping your daily calories low is often not the problem with a low carbohydrate diet. There is a tendency to not get enough calories because eating low carbohydrate foods usually means a low calorie count. In the beginning I had this problem, and I would always be tempted to eat more calories that had more carbohydrates in them. Eventually, I was able to find the right foods to maintain the daily calorie intake I needed. If you focus exclusively on carbohydrates, this can happen to you too. You need to keep your carbohydrate count within your set limits and still maintain the calorie count you desire. Although losing weight is healthy, losing weight quickly can be unhealthy.

## Portion size

I often hear people on television and read in books about portion size, especially as it relates to weight loss and nutrition, but with a type 2 diabetic, there are two important factors to consider when looking at the portion size. One is the percentage of carbohydrates to calories and the other is the self-discipline related to eating certain foods. Some foods may seem as if they are not high in carbohydrates and are low in calories as well. They should be perfect for a diabetic. But the serving size reveals the problem. An example is popcorn. One cup of popcorn has about six grams of carbohydrates and only 31 calories. This wouldn't be so bad if I had the self-discipline to eat only one cup of popcorn, but I don't think I have ever done this in my life. A serving for me would be more like four cups of popcorn. This would mean a total of 24 grams of carbohydrates and 124 calories. The total amount of carbohydrates is almost an entire meal for me and yet I have only eaten 124 calories. This is way too few calories to survive on. Type 2 diabetics need to avoid low calorie foods that are high in carbohydrates. This is not to say a small portion of popcorn can't be included in a diet, but it does take self-discipline.

## Exercise has a profound effect on glucose levels

The best exercise is the one that you are willing to do. My preferred exercise is walking. My second choice is swimming, but where I live, it is not an activity that can be done year round.

I have found that on the days that I walk the most, are the days when my glucose levels are the lowest. In fact, if I keep my carbohydrates to less than 100 grams and my daily intake of calories at approximately 2000, my blood sugar levels are as healthy as a non-diabetic, and my spikes in blood sugar are under 120. This is no different from a non-diabetic. This demonstrates the importance of exercise along with diet for a type 2 diabetic.

# Chapter 6

## Foods to Eat and Foods to Avoid

When I was growing up, they taught us about nutrition using the four food groups, and this is how I still see food in my diet. The groups were meat, dairy, cereal/grains, and fruits and vegetables. Unless you have additional medical issues and I do not, Type 2 diabetics can eat meat, most dairy, and vegetables. The entire cereal/grain group must be avoided as well as fruits. It is true that there is a lot of nutrition to be found in the groups that must be avoided, but this applies to those without type 2 diabetes.

## Cereals including brown rice and whole grains

Never mind what you hear from nutritionists about what

is healthy. Sure, whole grains are better than processed grains, but this does not apply to a type 2 diabetic. I ate a lot of white rice before my diagnosis, and during that time, I always heard people talking about how much better brown rice was to eat than white rice. After accepting the fact I was a diabetic I knew I couldn't eat white rice any more. One glucose test after a bowl of rice was all the information I needed to know. But is brown rice all right? The label on the back of rice tells you everything you need to know. Brown rice is clearly higher in fiber than white rice and 20 percent less in carbohydrates. The slight reduction in carbohydrates is not enough to help a type 2 diabetic. Brown rice is as dangerous as white rice. It is true that the higher fiber content makes brown rice more nutritional, but not for someone who has diabetes.

Regardless of whether someone is talking about rice, wheat, oats or any other grain, the issue of carbohydrates is the primary one for a diabetic. Whole grains sound like they are healthy, and they are for a non-diabetic; but you must choose your foods based upon how they affect your blood sugar first.

## Fruit

Fruit is another problem for the type 2 diabetic. Many of them are high in fiber and loaded with vitamins and minerals; they are also loaded with carbohydrates and must be avoided. Occasionally, a little fruit can be eaten, but the focus should be on those low in carbohydrates. Blackberries are among the lowest in carbohydrates, but even then portions must be kept small.

## Dairy foods

Almost everything dairy is fine with the exception of milk and yogurt. Anything else in the dairy group can usually be eaten, and you will be able to stay within a reasonable carbohydrate budget. Where I live there are low carbohydrate milks available as well as low carbohydrate yogurts. I don't use the milk often because I find that there is no cereal that is low enough in carbohydrates to use it on. The low carbohydrate yogurts only have four grams of carbohydrates and are available in a variety of flavors. I eat them often as a snack. These items may not be available in your area.

**Vegetables**

Almost all vegetables can be eaten, but there are a few exceptions. Although I consider corn to be a grain, many consider it a vegetable. Either way is bad for someone with type 2 diabetes. Potatoes also should be avoided. The other vegetables that are high in carbohydrates are most of the beans. With the exception of green beans, most beans are high in carbohydrates and should be avoided.

**Meat**

Almost all meat can be eaten. Although most meat has no carbohydrates, some of the processed meat may have a few carbohydrates. Examples of this include hot dogs and sausage. If you have a medical condition that does not allow red meat, you can focus your consumption on fish or poultry. These lean meats are healthy for you. I do not like fish, but I eat a lot of chicken. I also eat a lot of pork, especially at breakfast time.

**Read food labels**

Read food labels religiously. Never consume anything unless you have the information for both carbohydrates and calories. For foods without labels, look up the information. The Internet is a very good source for this, but there are also pocket guides you can carry around with you and use at home as well. Pay attention to serving size. What may seem to be a food lower in carbohydrates may not be lower at all. One food may have a serving size stated as one cup while another may be a half of a cup. Do not be fooled by marketing words on a package, claiming the product is healthy. Always remember that what may be very good for a non-diabetic, may be dangerous to a person who has type 2 diabetes.

# Chapter 7

## The importance of fiber in the diet

When I began a low carbohydrate diet, I had one side effect that became apparent quickly. To put it a delicately as possible, it was my bowels. At first it was a case of diarrhea that only lasted about 12 hours, but after this I was still having difficulty with loose bowels. I realized that I was most likely not getting enough fiber in my diet. My previous diet consisted of a lot of rice. Although terrible for a diabetic, rice made me regular, and I never had any problems. Switching to a low carbohydrate diet sent my fiber intake to low levels, and I felt it during my bowel movements.

You may experience this as well, but before you give up on a low carbohydrate intake, try consuming more vegetables. I now eat more vegetables than ever in my life. Some vegetables have a higher amount of fiber in them than others, and I try to focus on these. One the greatest sources of fiber in the world of vegetables are avocados. I love avocados. Although they are expensive, I eat at least a couple of them each week. Usually, I don't eat them with a recipe. I simply use a ripe, peeled avocado, then cut up and placed on a piece of deli meat. Served cold with mayonnaise, it is just like a sandwich, but without the bread. Other high fiber vegetables that I have grown fond of include spinach (raw), broccoli, cauliflower and celery.

## A word about fiber when counting carbohydrates

Fiber is that portion of the plant that cannot be digested. It moves through the digestive system and keeps everything moving forward inside the digestive system while absorbing excess water. For this reason, a diet high in fiber keeps a person regular and prevents loose bowels. The trouble with fiber is that it makes it tricky to count carbohydrates. The portions of carbohydrates that are fiber will not be digested, so it will not count when estimating your carbohydrate intakes. The question is how to factor in the grams of fiber in food.

Many will tell you that you can simply subtract the grams of fiber from the grams of carbohydrates. For example, if a serving of food has eight grams of carbohydrates and three grams of fiber, the amount of interest to you will be five grams of carbohydrates. This is often called the net carbohydrate count and can be seen on the packages of products that are marketed as low carbohydrate.

There are dieticians that say you should only subtract half

of the fiber content from the total carbohydrate count as long as it is a significant source of carbohydrates. This is usually defined as five grams of fiber or more. A third option is to ignore all of the fiber content when you calculate your daily carbohydrate intake and just add up the gross amount of carbohydrate grams. When doing this you will most likely be overstating your daily intake of carbohydrates; however, subtracting out the total amount of fiber may be underestimating carbohydrate intake.

Whatever you choose to do, make sure it is consistently done as you monitor your daily carbohydrates. As long as you calculate carbohydrates and fiber the same way each day, the only difference you will see is a specific target number for daily grams of carbohydrates. Although the daily target number may be higher or lower, depending upon the method used, a consistent approach will still lead to achieving the goal of glucose level reduction.

I can attest to the effect that foods high in fiber have on my body. Avocado is a perfect example. One cup of sliced avocado has approximately 12 grams of carbohydrates; this is somewhat high to include in my diet. But the fiber content in this same cup is 10 grams. When I eat avocados, there is little effect on my glucose level, so I can only conclude that there is a net carbohydrate content that needs to be counted. In this case it would be 12-10 which is only a small two grams of carbohydrates.

## A word about low carbohydrate recipes

There are many people who are type 2 diabetics that have recipes you can try. They can be found in books, on the Internet and maybe even from friends. Some of these recipes are designed for type 2 diabetics, but others are for those people who follow a low carbohydrate diet. Some of these people take a low carbohydrate diet to an extreme that may not be appropriate. I have read of people who are on a diet of less than 20 grams of carbohydrates a day. If this is required for your diabetic condition and a doctor has recommended it, by all means follow your doctor's advice. For most type 2 diabetics, there is only a need to reduce carbohydrate levels enough to get glucose levels under control.

In the beginning, getting your diabetes under control is the priority and not a tasty recipe. Although I am experimenting with different recipes now, at first I focused on eating low carbohydrate foods and lowering glucose levels. If this meant eating a ham and cheese sandwich with no bread, then that is what I did. Lowering your blood sugar is too important to mess around with recipes. Save that for after you get your glucose levels down.

# Chapter 8

## No more sweets?

Ideally, you should not be eating any sweets. But I can't resist, and you may not be able to either. I am a big coffee drinker, and the first thing I missed on a low carbohydrate diet was a pastry or donut with my coffee. At least, a few cookies with my coffee would be nice. This was no longer possible. Never mind the sugar content, the carbohydrates were entirely too high for my daily limits. Even with sugar free cookies, the carbohydrate count is often too high. I have found the solution to be with a narrow group of sweets that are lower in carbohydrates than most. This combined with portion size and I am able to squeeze in a little treat now and then.

An example of these sweets is M&M's peanut candies. Each candy has approximately 1.1 grams of carbohydrates. By eating a maximum of eight candies, I am consuming approximately nine grams of carbohydrates with less than 90 calories. They come in small packets containing seven or eight peanut candies. This is perfect for me because it represents a perfect serving size I can fit into my diet. It is usually cheaper to buy a large bag of these candies such as one pound, but I do not have the discipline to only eat eight of them out of a large bag. I can exercise enough discipline to limit myself to eating only a small packet. It is difficult, but I can do it.

Other possible sweets for my diet are half of a low carbohydrate flour tortilla with a teaspoon of sugar free jam. I also will consume one or two squares of dark chocolate. In general, dark chocolate offers many possibilities. I recently bought these cookie sticks stuffed with dark chocolate. On the outside, they are about half the size of a taquito, but they only have six carbohydrates and 45 calories. Right now, I only eat one per day. What all of these sweet snacks have in common is that they are all under 10 carbohydrates. And I limit myself to only one serving each day, so I can stay within my daily carbohydrate budget.

# Chapter 9

## Eating out at restaurants

My eating behavior is dictated by my glucose testing. If I find that I am spiking too high in my glucose levels, I have to modify my eating strategy. This is the same way I approach restaurants. Many restaurant chains have their nutritional information online, and most of them have information printed that can be used at the restaurant before ordering. Over time, I have developed certain strategies for certain restaurants, but these are general ideas that I follow that may be helpful to you.

## Burger Joints

I have found that I can eat hamburgers and cheeseburgers, but no bun. There are a few carbohydrates in ketchup, but my body seems to be able to handle this. I can't eat french fries. Although I probably could steal a couple of fries from the person I am eating with, I don't have the self-discipline to eat two french fries, so no fries for me.

## Mexican fast food

I have a great difficulty eating at fast food Mexican restaurants. Many get tacos and burritos at lunchtime or for a quick dinner, but I can't eat a lot of refried beans and even less rice. These are common ingredients at most Mexican restaurants. Add to this, the tortillas are not good for me. When I am with other people who are eating at a fast food restaurant like this, I will usually order soft tacos and lay them out flat to eat everything but the tortilla. Chicken is a good choice of meat. With careful eating, I can keep the carbohydrates low, but chances are I will not get enough to eat.

## Pizza

I can eat everything but the crust; unfortunately the crust

is usually very high in carbohydrates. What I will do is eat the top of the pizza with a fork. This includes all of the cheese, sauce and the toppings. I have found that my glucose levels will not spike high if I only eat one medium or two small slices of pizza when it is thin crust, but I never eat the outer portion of the crust.

**Chinese food**

I can't eat fried rice or the noodles, but that still leaves me with a few low carbohydrate dishes. I love Kung Pao chicken and am fond of chicken and broccoli as well. My glucose levels do not spike high with these foods.

It takes time to know what you can eat and not eat when eating out. Often you must rely on glucose testing to know how your body will react. In the beginning, when you are attempting to bring down your glucose levels, you should probably avoid eating out. Focus on the foods you have a good carbohydrate number for and get your glucose numbers down. Once you have decided to attempt eating at a restaurant, it may be best to keep your portions small. Naturally, what counts the most is the glucose reading approximately 1 ½ hours after you have eaten your meal.

## How I survived a breakfast buffet

My favorite meal of the day is breakfast, and my favorite place to eat breakfast is a buffet. Here, in Las Vegas, we have some of the best breakfast buffets anybody would ever want. As a type 2 diabetic, this was a big problem for me; however, I have learned to circumvent this problem. The first thing I decided was to eliminate my syrup plate. This was a plate of food I would get that consisted of pancakes, waffles and French toast. All of which I covered with syrup. The carbohydrates on this plate alone would today most likely give me a stroke. I decided to eliminate the pastries at the end of my meal such as a donut, tart and Danish. This still left me with two or three plates of food. I cut back to a very small portion of hash browns and loaded up on more eggs, bacon and sausage. I also had an omelet and my favorite Mexican food: chorizo. Even though most of the foods were low in carbohydrate, the quantity added up fast and an hour and a half after I finished eating my sugar level hit 168. Although this number is high, I'm scared to think what it used to be before my diagnosis. Now, months later, I have been exercising regularly, and I am able to keep my sugar spike to the high 150s. I have also cut back on the portion sizes a bit and of course, I don't eat at the buffet every day. It is only a treat for me every few weeks.

# Chapter 10

## Is the damage from type 2 diabetes reversible?

Generally speaking, it is not. This is especially true with the nerve damage to the legs. However, there is evidence that the progression of the damage to your body can be halted. The condition of neuropathy that I experienced has not gotten any worse since I was able to get my glucose under control.

There are advertisements you may read and hear that claim to reverse neuropathy, but I would be highly skeptical. Focus on stopping further damage to your body, and then you can experience for yourself how your body is reacting to a low carbohydrate diet.

# Can type 2 diabetes be prevented?

Many of you reading this may not have type 2 diabetes but have a parent or sibling that does. This will naturally bring up the thought about getting type 2 diabetes yourself at some time in the future. The research done in this area has been inconclusive; much more needs to be done. Like other diseases, there does seem to be a strong genetic component to it, so if one or more of your blood relatives has type 2 diabetes, you may develop it yourself. This is especially true if a parent has had or has the disease. What may be true is that an individual has a genetic predisposition to type 2 diabetes. Although the majority of people on a high carbohydrate diet will never develop the disease, those who have a family history of it, may have a higher probability of becoming type 2 diabetics. If this is true, then a diet that is lower in carbohydrates could prevent a person from developing type 2 diabetes. I stress the word "could" because at this time, there is no way of knowing if this is true. Even so, by eliminating most of the sugary snacks and desserts from your diet and switching to whole grains instead of processed grains will only make you healthier. Keep your weight down and exercise daily; you will be better off for it regardless of any genetic predisposition to type 2 diabetes.

# A Last Word

After you find out that you have type 2 diabetes, you may want to live in denial. I did this for a few days, but I was able to snap out of it. If you have recently been diagnosed, you may not be in a state of denial, but you may be feeling depressed. This is also a natural reaction. Maybe you are someone who has been aware of their diabetic condition for quite some time, but you simply can't take the steps needed to control your glucose. Whatever your situation is, if you are a type 2 diabetic and do not have your glucose levels under control, you need to begin doing so right now. Do not put it off until tomorrow.

# Resources to Help You with Type 2 Diabetes

## The American Diabetes Association

The American Diabetes Association is a non-profit organization that is dedicated to help as many people as they can with both type 1 and type 2 diabetes. The work they do is for the benefit of society in general and individuals as well.

The number of diabetics in the American population is almost nine percent, and many of these people do not know what to do about their condition. The ADA offers assistance in many ways. One of the most important ways they can help is with information, but simply knowing you are not alone is a great source of emotional support.

The ADA has information that can help a diabetic at every stage of their life and can aid in increasing the quality of life and increase the chances of living a longer life. The information they have is provided by mail, email and even the smart phone. Text messages can be sent to remind a diabetic to take required medication and smartphone apps exist to help with the proper diet.

**American Diabetes Association – type 2 diabetes information:**

http://www.diabetes.org/diabetes-basics/type-2/

**WebMD**

WebMD is one of the most popular and authoritative websites for medical information on the Internet. Their section on type 2 diabetes is very good.

http://www.webmd.com/diabetes/guide/type-2-diabetes-resources

# About the Author

Matthew Lashley is a writer and indie publisher who lives in Las Vegas, Nevada. Since his diagnosis of type 2 diabetes and subsequent success at getting it under control, he continues to keep it under control with diet, exercise and medication.

# Other publications from Teela Books

## Sports and Horse Racing Betting Systems That Work! by Ken Osterman

The book contains some of the best sports betting systems from Ken Osterman. These are systems that he has used himself successfully at both racetracks and sports books. The rules for each system are clearly explained and the systems are explained clearly so it is understood why they work. Tips for improving these systems are also provided.

There are 10 systems in this book that cover horse racing,

football and baseball. Here is a list of the systems with the sport that is covered and the title of the system.

Horse racing

Quarter Horse - The Hidden Speed Horse Angle

Thoroughbred - Best Jockey – Long shot Method

Thoroughbred - Bet the Fastest Horse

Thoroughbred - Show a profit down under

Harness - The qualifier advantage

Harness - Morning Line Overlay

Sports Betting

NFL Football - The Injured Star

NFL Football - The Hat Trick

Baseball - The AAA Surprise

Baseball - The Underdog Advantage


This book is currently available:

In Kindle format on Amazon:

http://www.amazon.com/dp/B00JTMWDNM


It is also available on iBooks, Barnes & Noble, Kobo, Inktera, Scribd, 24Symbols, and Tolino.


It is also available in Paperback on Amazon

http://www.amazon.com/dp1507800142

# The Path to Harness Racing Handicapping Profits by Douglas Masters

## The Secrets of Harness Race Profits Revealed!

This book represents three decades of handicapping and betting harness races and is a summary of observations that are important to being a winning player. This book summarizes the conclusions on what made the author a winning player. There is no magic formula to become a winning player and the author is the first to say that there is more than one road to profits. This book is the road taken by Doug Masters to becoming a winning player. Becoming a winning player is part art and part skill, so it is impossible to summarize it as a mechanical method; however, Doug attempts to outline his process in the second half of the book.

This book may be difficult for beginning harness handicappers to read because it does not explain any basic terminology. There are, however, glossaries of harness racing terms online as well in the racing programs of harness tracks.

There are no winning examples in this book.

This is a quote from the author in the introduction.

"You will find no past performances listed in this book; this is intentional. Anyone who has been around harness racing for even a few years has probably read various books and publications offering a handicapping system. All of them will have examples of how a handicapping system or angle picked a winner. Anyone can do this, especially when so many of these authors are working backwards from the winner. To me, it is simply a waste of time. And besides, only a mediocre or inexperienced handicapper is going to believe there is a single path to success in wagering. This book consists of my observations of the sport and how it relates to my own handicapping perspective. If you are looking for a system that represents some sort of absolute truth, you're looking in the wrong place."

Topics include: Handicapping Factors, Drivers, Horse Form, Speed, Pace, Class, Post position, Track, Statistics, Betting multiple racetracks.

This book is currently available:

In Kindle format on Amazon:

http://www.amazon.com/dp/B00I5B13MU

It is also available on iBooks, Barnes & Noble, Kobo, Inktera, Scribd, 24Symbols, and Tolino.

It is also available in Paperback on Amazon

http://www.amazon.com/dp/1508707553

# Type 2 Diabetes: From diagnosis to a new way of life by Matthew Lashley

From the author

This book tells the story of how my diabetic condition was discovered, my denial of the condition, then the work done to get my glucose level to levels that are close to normal. There is no magic solution to treating type 2 diabetes, but I hope the information that I gathered and applied to my own life may be helpful to everyone struggling with type 2 diabetes. There is no cure, and I will have this condition the rest of my life. However, type 2 diabetes can be treated and controlled with the proper approach and lifestyle changes. You can have a better quality of life with a diet that is compatible with this disease.

Topics include:

From denial to self-blame

How I found out what type 2 diabetes was

Acceptance and getting down to work

Medication

Type 2 diabetes is a serious illness

How many carbohydrates per day should the limit be?

My target glucose levels

Foods to eat and foods to avoid

The importance of fiber in the diet

Eating out at restaurants

Is the damage from type 2 diabetes reversible?

Can type 2 diabetes be prevented?

This book is currently available:

In Kindle format on Amazon:

http://www.amazon.com/dp/B00IRJ9L1K

It is also available on iBooks, Barnes & Noble, Kobo, Inktera, Scribd, 24Symbols, and Tolino.

It is also available in Paperback on Amazon

http://www.amazon.com/dp/1508826005

# The Quick and Dirty NFL Football Handicapping Method by Ken Osterman

The purpose of this book is to explain a fundamental approach to making a profit betting on professional football games, especially for those with little time to handicap them.

This method will help you find an overlay in the point spread using the simplest and quickest method possible.

The Quick and Dirty NFL Football Handicapping Method teaches you how to create your own point spread for each game in the NFL.

Table of Contents

Introduction

An important first step in becoming a winning bettor

The basis of the Quick and Dirty NFL Method

How to create your own point spread

NFL 2013 season Week 7 - Miami Dolphins at Buffalo Bills

NFL 2013 season Week 9 - Tampa Bay Buccaneers at

Seattle Seahawks

NFL 2013 season Week 15 - Baltimore Ravens at Detroit Lions

Money Management

Improving this method

Mistakes to Avoid

Conclusion

This book is currently available:

In Kindle format on Amazon:

http://www.amazon.com/dp/B00NX9X81I

It is also available on iBooks, Barnes & Noble, Kobo, Inktera, Scribd, 24Symbols, and Tolino.

It is also available in Paperback on Amazon

http://www.amazon.com/dp/151202614X

**Betting on Major League Baseball**

**The Underdog Method by Ken Osterman**

The essence of any good baseball handicapping system is to find games to bet on that will result in long-term profits. In other words, finding overlays. The Underdog Method uses an approach to not only find these good bets, but does so by creating a money line that can be compared to the one offered by sports books.

Author and sports gambler, Ken Osterman, explains this system in an easy-to-understand way, and then uses an entire day of baseball games as examples. Each game is handicapped per the rules of the Underdog Method, and then a betting line is created. This line is compared to a specific sports book's money line. It is then decided, based upon specific rules, whether a good bet exists or not.

Although demonstrating the effectiveness of any betting system is limited in a book, the approach to Major League Baseball betting using the Underdog System is significantly different than the simple angles and methods seen elsewhere.

This book is currently available:

In Kindle format on Amazon:

http://www.amazon.com/dp/B01220NL8I

It is also available on iBooks, Barnes & Noble, Kobo, Inktera, Scribd, 24Symbols, and Tolino.

It is also available in Paperback on Amazon

http://www.amazon.com/dp/1515180646

# Free Things To Do on the Las Vegas Strip
# A Self-Guided Tour by Matt Lashley

The Strip is world famous and not only for the casinos, but also for the many things to see and do. Of course, a lot of what you can do here costs money, but there are a number of things to do that are free.

This book is a self-guided tour, taking you step by step down the Strip to visit all of the notable free things to do. This excludes most of the photo opportunities, because the entire length of the strip is filled with places to take a photo of you, your friends and relatives. Only a few places of interest, directly in our travel path, are mentioned. Also, shopping sites have been excluded except for three unique stores of interest on the Strip.

The trip begins at the Welcome to Fabulous Las Vegas sign and ends in the downtown portion of Las Vegas Blvd. This is the old section of Las Vegas and is not considered a part of the Strip. I have included it to provide a complete Las Vegas experience.

This book is currently available:

In Kindle format on Amazon:

http://www.amazon.com/dp/B01EW6DWXY

It is also available on iBooks, Barnes & Noble, Kobo, Inktera, Scribd, 24Symbols, and Tolino.

It is also available in Paperback on Amazon

http://www.amazon.com/dp/1533524084

**Stealth Betting Systems for Winning at Casinos by Luke Meadows**

Stop Losing and Start Winning in Las Vegas casinos!

Author and casino gambler, Luke Meadows, explains his betting methods he uses in Las Vegas casinos in an easy-to-understand way. There are casino systems for the games of roulette, craps, blackjack, Let It Ride, and Keno. Mr. Meadows is convinced that your best chance of winning is small wins using smart gambling systems, and to do this without bringing attention to yourself – a stealth mode of casino gambling.

In all of this time Luke, like most of us, has experienced both winning and losing. Over time, his trips to Las Vegas have produced more profits than losses. The reason for this is his method of gambling at casinos. A method that he has honed and fine-tuned to the point where he has the best chance of winning, while at the same time, keeping his losses low.

This book is currently available:

In Kindle format on Amazon:

http://www.amazon.com/dp/B01KGSN63S

It is also available on iBooks, Barnes & Noble, Kobo, Inktera, Scribd, 24Symbols, and Tolino.

It is also available in Paperback on Amazon

http://www.amazon.com/dp/1537175939

For the latest information about our publications, along with articles by some of our authors, please

visit our website at


http://www.teela-books.com

www.ingramcontent.com/pod-product-compliance
Lightning Source LLC
Chambersburg PA
CBHW070600290526
45790CB00002B/740